Natural Winter Care
20 Recipes for Your Healthy Skin and Hair

Table of Contents

Introduction

Winter can be rough...

The cold air and dry climate in the winter can ravage your skin and hair. It can cause your skin to feel stretched out and, in some cases, crack. The winter environment can make your skin flake as well. Your hair can dry out, frizz, and the ends can split. Dried out hair can also fly away due to static electricity caused by just brushing your hair.

Getting ready for winter means more than just boosting your immune system and weather-proofing your car and home. It also means having the tools necessary to protect your skin and hair from drying out and being damaged. This book can give you the tools to do that. This book contains advice and recipes to help keep your hair and skin healthy and free from damage. What are you waiting for?

Chapter 1 – The colder months and you

As the temperature drops, we change out our clothes, putting the summer wardrobe away and taking out the long sleeves and sweaters. We call the heating and air guys to check our furnace, and we take our vehicles to the shop to winterize them. We mow our lawns one last time and put lime on it so it's ready for the first mowing of the new year. We make sure we have enough wood for the fireplace and even double check the insulation in the attic.

We go to the doctor for check-ups, and some of us get flu shots, but we overlook the two things we struggle with throughout the winter, our hair and skin.

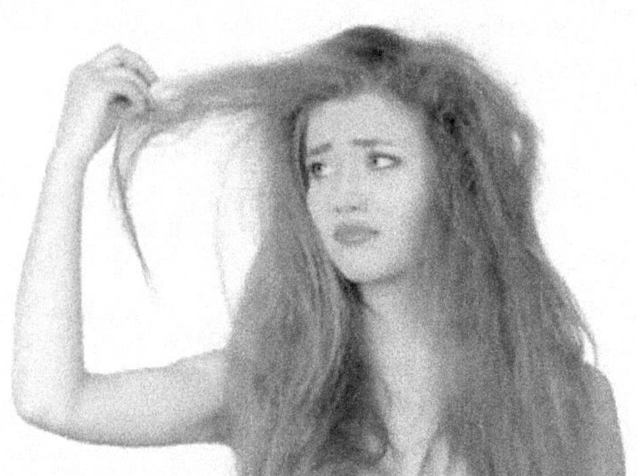

Colder air and chapped skin...

Your lips aren't the only things drying out and chapping. Winter air is cold and dry. There is often little to no moisture in the air that whips around outside.

It can also make your skin contract and dry out. This makes your skin feel tight and crack. If you are prone to eczema and psoriasis, you will be more prone to rashes that turn raw, crack, and even bleed in some cases.

Couple this with the heater and/or fireplace going on in your home and your skin is miserable all winter long.

Cold air and artificial heat dries any moisture in the air. This moisture is what your skin absorbs on a daily basis to keep its elasticity. Your hair is no different.

During the winter, your hair is constantly trying to get the moisture it needs from its roots, but the stalk and ends of the hair are dry due to the environment outside and the one we make inside to keep us warm and toasty.

It's more inclined to break and split, not to mention fly off in all directions when we brush it because of static electricity. We go to the salon and have it trimmed of the damage and even ask for a treatment for it, but your hair doesn't stay pristine for long during the winter, and you want to find a way to keep the damage under control to prevent your wallet from feeling the strain.

Some basic things you can do...
Staying hydrated doesn't stop when the thermometer dips. If anything, it's just as important to stay hydrated in the winter as it is in the summer. Water and coconut water can help with this perfectly.

You can add a couple of ounces of coconut water to the juice you drink in the morning to give an extra kick of electrolytes.

This may sound funny, but those hot baths we love to take in the winter actually dry out our skin. Luke warm to cool baths are the key to keeping your skin hydrated from the outside. I know it's unheard of to take cool baths in the winter, but it will help keep your skin moisturized.

If you just can't bring yourself to take those cool to warm baths, air dry in your room. This will give your skin the time it needs to adsorb the moisture of the bath or shower you just got through taking.

Finding a light moisturizer to put on your skin while you are still damp will help your skin as well. Lotion, baby oil, or other moisturizer will help to keep in the moisture. It will also help keep your skin soft and prevent drying.

Your hair is an even greater challenge. If you use styling tools, you dry out your hair more readily than others who don't. Conditioners can help, but your hair needs back-up. Let it dry naturally instead of hitting it with a blow-dryer. Doing these at least once a week can help.

Chapter 2 – Vitamins and herbal supplements

There is always talk and speculation on whether vitamins and minerals taken internally actually help skin and hair stay healthy. They do, but you may have to up the amount you're already taking or add herbal supplements targeted at keeping your skin and hair healthy.

Aloe

One cannot talk about skin without bringing this plant. This is one of the most widely used herbs for dry and rough skin. It can also help repair cracked and raw skin.

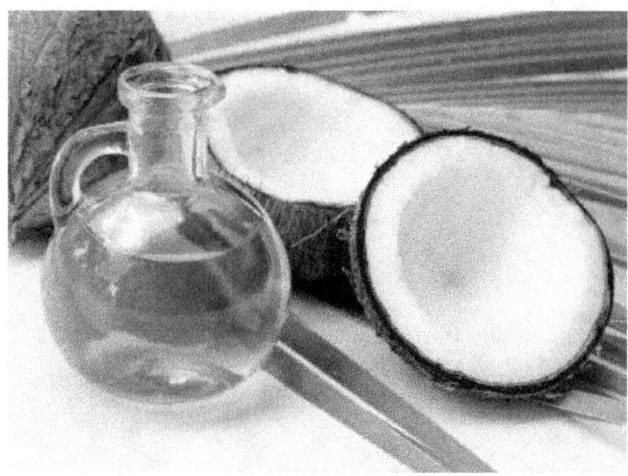

Coconut oil

When it comes to moisture, coconut oil is king. You can directly apply it to your skin for immediate relief, make it into an ointment for spot treatments, and even apply it to hair to tame frizz and prevent split ends and breaking.

Jojoba oil

This, along with coconut oil, come closest to the natural sebum your scalp produces to moisturize your hair. Just like coconut oil, it can be applied in small amounts to wet or dry hair to tame frizz, moisturize hair at the root and ends, and prevent splitting and breaking.

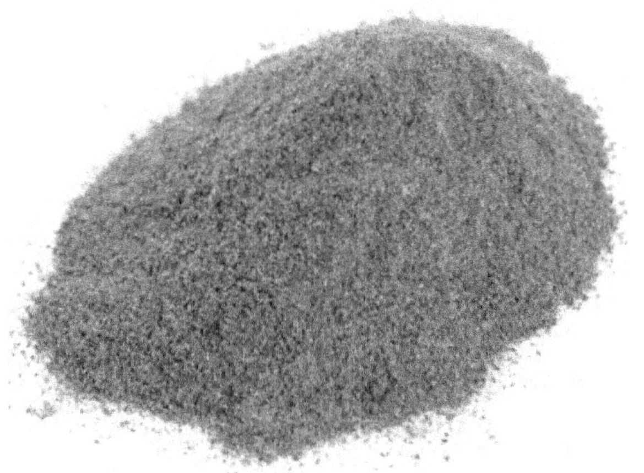

Horsetail

This is an herb you can take in capsule form or drink as a tea. It keeps your skin healthy and your hair strong and resistant to splitting and breaking. Horsetail can even strengthen your hair.

Humidifiers and Vaporizers

These are the best ways to combat the lack of humidity in your home due to running heaters and having your fireplace going. They can replace the lost moisture in your home, reducing the chance for static electricity.

Kelp

This seaweed has been used in facial masks and mineral baths. The vitamins and minerals in this food can keep your skin glowing and healthy, prevent your hair from breaking and even strengthen your hair at the root. Used as an ingredient in mineral baths, it can sooth rough skin and help to repair the damage the cold air can do to it.

Lavender Flowers

This flower and its essential oil are highly recommended in returning moisture and repairing skin. It is often added to lotions, herbal baths, body oils, and sugar scrubs.

Lotions

There are a multitude of lotions on the market, but many either leave your skin greasy or they feel like you haven't even applied them to your skin. Finding the right balance can be a pain. The best course of action would be to find a good lotion base and add your own essential oils to insure you're getting the moisture you need.

Oatmeal baths

These are a good way to restore lost moisture in the skin. You can combine baking soda and borax as well as essential oils and herbs to further soften and moisturize the skin.

Retinol vs Beta Carotene...

Both are vitamin A, but which one is better? Retinol is fat soluble and your body stores what it can't use when you take more than you should. This often leads to vitamin A toxicity.

To avoid this, switch to Beta Carotene. Your body changes this into vitamin A as your body needs it to keep your skin soft and your hair healthy. It also can help with keep your eyes healthy as well.

Spirulina

A superfood most people add to smoothies, this is packed with many vitamins and minerals your skin and hair needs to stay healthy.

Vitamin C

Another anti-oxidant, this vitamin is a wonder when it comes to helping your skin's elasticity and healthy glow.

Vitamin E and Selenium

You can use the liquid E to repair damaged skin, but you can help prevent your skin from getting damaged by taking the vitamin internally. The selenium helps boost the action of the vitamin to make it more effective.

Chapter 3 – Essential oils

There are many essential oils which can be used in baths, oils, and lotions to help keep your skin and hair smooth, soft, and moisturized.

Chamomile, Roman

This is mainly for the skin. It can help soothe the irritation caused by harsh winds and cold temperatures. It can also aid in ridding your skin of rough spots and rashes. It also helps speed healing for dry and damaged skin.

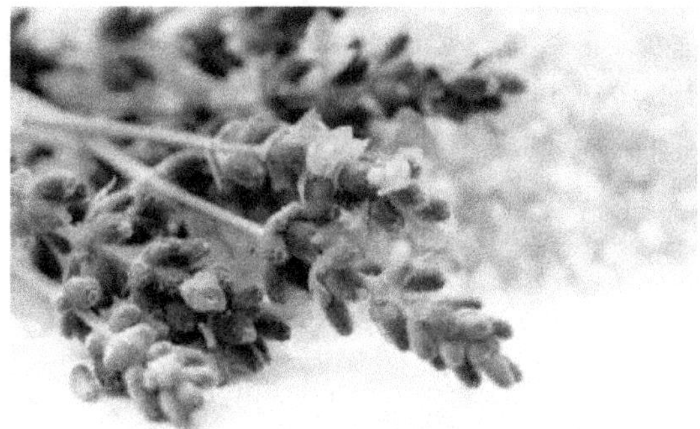

Lavender

I am including this here as an essential oil, because it is not only the most widely used, but the most highly recommended essential oil for skin conditions. It can stop itching, repair skin damage, and even treat rashes when added to base oils and put in lip balms and ointments. You can also incorporate it into sugar scrubs.

Geranium

Your skin itches, turns an ashy pale, and gets irritated when exposed to cold air. Geranium can soothe the itching response, helping the body speed healing and soothe the skin.

Base oils

You can't talk about essential oils without mentioning base or carrier oils. You should never apply essential oils to the skin without diluting them first. Doing so can cause contact dermatitis. Always dilute your essential oils no matter the grade, just to be safe.

Apricot seed oil

This is a widely used, multi-purpose oil. It is light enough to use on its own without mixing it with other carrier oils and is often a substitute for Sweet Almond oil.

Beeswax

More a wax than an oil, it is used to make ointments and body/lip balms for its healing properties.

Coco Butter

Though a solid wax, it is combined with coconut and other oils for body balms, lip balms and ointments for its moisturizing properties.

Coconut oil

This was mentioned in the previous chapter. It is often used in ointments and lips balms to treat chapped skin.

Grapeseed oil

This is a carrier oil which can be added to lighter oils to promote healing and moisture in the skin. It has antioxidant properties and has little to no fragrance of its own.

Jojoba oil

This was discussed in the previous chapter and is more a wax than an oil. It can be mixed with lighter oils to promote healing and keep moisture in the skin.

Sweet Almond Oil

This is the most popular carrier oil in aromatherapy. It is light, odor-free, and very versatile. It contains many of the vitamins your body needs to combat drying and chapping.

Virgin Olive Oil

This carrier oil is high in vitamin E. This is the first pressing of the olives, and has a pungent olive fragrance. It is used in small amounts and mixed with lighter oils.

Chapter 4 – Your face

We can cover most of our body before going out into the cold for work or running errands, but your face often takes the brunt of cold winds and harsh weather. If your face goes without moisture, it will show it by chapped lips, stretched skin, and wrinkles.

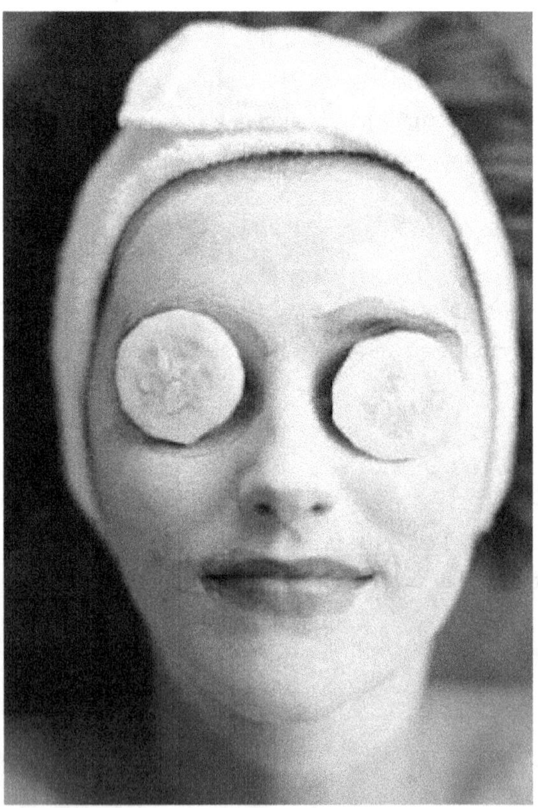

Moisturizers

You can get these in most stores, but to better protect your skin, you're going to need something to put on your skin before you go out and before you go to bed after you cleanse your face.

Facial masks

These are best done when the day is over. It will help to condition your facial skin and return the moisture lost by the whipping winds and cold temps.

Seaweed Mask

DRY INGREDIENTS

3 tbsp ground Kelp

3 tbsp ground Spirulina

OILS

2 tbsp Sweet Almond or Apricot oil

1 tsp Grapseed oil

1 tsp jojoba oil

10 Drops Lavender Essential oil

5 Drops Geranium Essential oil

3 Drops Roman Chamomile Essential oi

- Mix the dry ingredients and set side.

- In a dark glass bottle, mix the oils well.

- Take 2 tablespoons of the dry ingredients and moisten them into a paste by using luke warm water

- Add 8 drops of the oil to the mask mixture

- Apply to your face evenly and allow it to dry. Avoid the eyes, nostrils, and mouth area.

- You can remoisten it the mask to remove it.

- Follow it up by taking a cotton ball and placing Grapeseed oil on it.

- Apply the grapeseed oil to the face lightly.

  o This will help lock in the nutrients you just put into your skin.

  o It will also help moisturize your facial skin as well.

Lavender Mask

DRY INGREDIENTS

1/4 cup ground Lavender Flowers

1/4 Cup ground oats

WET INGREDIENTS

1/8 Cup of pure Aloe Juice

3 tbsp Sweet Almond or Apricot seed oil

1 tsp Grapeseed oil

1/4 tsp Virgin Olive oil

10 Drops of Geranium Essential Oil

8 Drops of Roman Chamomile Essential Oil

- Mix the dry ingredients

- Gently warm the Aloe to Skin temperature

- Add the aloe to 3 tablespoons of the oats and Lavender Flower mixture until it forms a paste

- Add 8 Drops of the oils and mix again.

- Place evenly on the face, being careful to avoid the areas listed in the first mask.

- Leave until dry and remoisten to remove.

- Use Grapeseed oil to further moisturize the face.

Quick moisture oil

1 tbsp Sweet Almond or Apricot Seed oil

1 tsp Jojoba Oil

4 Drops of Lavender Essential oi

3 Drops of Roman Chamomile Essential oil

- Mix together well and apply to the face with a cotton ball.

- Avoid the nostrils and eye area.

To add a little punch to your nightly moisturizer, add 6 drops of Lavender Essential oil per tablespoon of moisturizer used.

You can do the same to your morning moisturizer as well.

Morning Juice

What you put in your body is just as important as what you put on it to protect your skin.

2 Medium Carrots

1 Medium Orange

1 Medium Red Apple

- Run all ingredients through a juicer and enjoy.

- You can also put these in a smoothie with a banana and 1/4 cup of Mango and 1/4 cup of Avocado.

Lip Balm

2 tbsp beeswax beads

2 tbsp coconut oil

1 1/2 tbsp jojoba oil

1/2 tbsp coco butter

20 Drops of Peppermint essential oil (another good oil for the skin)

10 Drops of Lavender essential oil

- Place all the oils in a double boiler until all are melted

- Add the essential oil when the mixture is still warm. Mix well.

- Pour the mixture into lip balm containers.

- If it is too soft, use 1 tbsp of both jojoba and coco butter.

- Apply as needed to condition and moisturize lips.

Chapter 5 – Your hair

With blow drying, flat and curling irons, hairspray and all the other things you do to it to make road-worthy, it goes through a lot of abuse. Conditioners are a mixed bag, with some being too heavy and some to light. They are mildly effective, but most are rinsed off before you step out the shower.

Protein Pack

4 Egg yolks, raw and scrambled

1/2 tsp Kelp

1/2 tsp Horsetail

2 tbsp Apple Cider vinegar

1/2 cup hot water

2 cups of water

- Boil the 1/2 cup of water and add the herbs.
- Let the herbs steep for 10 minutes before straining.
- Mix the 2 cups of water with the Apple Cider Vinegar
- When the water is warm, put 3 tbsp of the tea in the egg.
- Place the egg mixture in your hair for twenty minutes
- Rinse with the Apple Cider mixture
- Wash as normal

The protein from the eggs and the nutrients from the herbs will reconditions the hair. The Apple Cider Vinegar mixture will make sure all the eggs washes out of the hair, taking any build up from styling products with it. If you need to, repeat the Apple Cider Vinegar mix until the hair is rinsed. The ACV will rebalance the HP on the scalp.

You can also use the ACV mixture as an after-rinse to your normal routine to prevent build-up of the styling products.

You can add essential oils to the ACV mix, but you have to add 12 drops directly to the ACV before you add the water to make sure the essential oils mix properly.

Making your own shampoo
Yes, you can make your own shampoo and only have the ingredients you want in it according to your hair type and control frizz better than buying all those products that tout frizz control.

Where does frizz come from?
Frizz happens when the hair is devoid of the moisture and proteins it needs to retain its moisture. Using harsh products on the hair, shampooing too often, bitter cold, and running the heater can all contribute to dry hair and frizz. Not getting nutrients on a daily basis can cause your hair to become brittle as well. Two of the major causes of extremely dry and brittle hair are perming and coloring. Both of these can leave the hair dry, brittle, prone to frizzing and breaking.

Homemade shampoo

4 oz Doctor Bronner's castille soap

2 of carrier oil

distilled water

1 tsp of an essential oil blend (You can pre-mix this.)

- Shred the bar of soap.

    o I recommend Doctor Bronner's unscented or aloe soap bar. Doctor Bronner's lacks all the phosphorous and other ingredients which are not necessary for cleaning the hair and scalp.

- Place the shreds in a blender

- Add the carrier oil of your choice

    o I am going to include oil combinations below.

- Turn the blender on medium speed as you add the water.

    o You want enough water to make it soapy but still be able to pour out of an existing shampoo bottle.

- Lastly, add the essential oil blend.

- Put the blender on liquify for two minutes and then pour into a clean and empty existing shampoo bottle.

Since this is a natural shampoo, you need to keep two things in mind:

1. You will have to shake it if you do not use it for a couple of days. It will separate due to lack of binders/emulsifiers.

2. It will not lather as much as you expect to. This is due to the lack of phosphorous and other ingredients designed to make shampoo foam.

<u>*Oil combinations for the shampoo*</u>

EXTREMELY DRY AND DAMAGED HAIR

1/2 ounce Virgin Olive Oil

1/2 ounce Jojoba oil

1/2 ounce Grapeseed oil

1/2 ounce Sweet Almond or Apricot seed oil

It will deeply condition the hair while you are shampooing with it. Once in the hair, leave the shampoo in the hair while you soap the rest of your body.

Rinse with purified water or an ACV and water mixture. Believe it or not, ACV and water helps to tame tangles and frizz. The down side is that your hair will smell like salad dressing.

DRY AND FRIZZED HAIR

1 ounce of Sweet Almond Oil

1/2 ounce of Coconut oil

1/2 ounce of Jojoba oil

This combination provides more vitamin E and conditioners while you are shampooing. If you want to leave the shampoo, you can.

WINTER GUARD SHAMPOO

4 ounces of Doctor Bronner's Aloe Soap

1/2 ounce of Coconut oil

1/2 Ounce of Jojoba Oil

4 ounces of Lavender and Chamomile Tea

1/4 tsp Geranium essential oil

1/4 tsp Rosemary essential oil (Scalp and hair conditioning)

1/2 tsp Lavender essential oil

COLD WEATHER SHAMPOO

4 Ounces of Doctor Bronner's Peppermint Soap Bar

2 Ounces of Jojoba oil

1/2 tsp of Lavender essential oil

1/4 tsp Rosemary essential oil

1/4 tsp Roman Chamomile essential oil

Frizz fix

Sometimes, even with all the treatment and care you have to preventing frizz and fly-away strands, you will still get frustrated while brushing or styling your hair.

1/4 cup Jojoba oil

1/4 Cup coconut oil

1/4 tsp Lavender essential oil

1/4 tsp Geranium essential oil

- Melt the coconut oil in a double boiler
- Add the Jojoba oil
- Mix the essential oils
- When the Jojoba and coconut oil are Luke warm, add the essential oils.
- Place in a reusable bottle.
- Place small amount in your hands.
- Rub your hands together and apply to either moist hair before drying or on dry hair to spot treat frizz.

Chapter 6 – From the neck down...

You have a lot more skin than just the skin on your face. Your body takes abuse from the heaters and cold, bitter air, too. Your skin is your first line of protection against injury, infection, and illness. It is, quite literally, the largest organ of your body, and when it's not healthy, it shows.

Showering or taking baths with hot water may feel good when you're cold, but it can dry out your skin just as fast as stepping outside on a bitter cold day without protection. You boil and blanche your vegetables in hot water. Your bath water may not be that hot, but it's hot enough to open pores and allow dirt and other things to settle in its pores.

As you dry your skin from taking a hot bath, it becomes tight. This is because it's drying out. I suggested a couple of ways to prevent this in the previous chapter, but here are some recipes you can mix at home to help you moisturize your skin during and after your bathing or showering.

Mineral baths

This can add moisture to your skin as you bathe. The combination of borax (a natural mineral) and baking soda (sodium bicarbonate) along with salts or oatmeal can soothe the skin and make it soft and bring back its elasticity.

Basic Mineral Bath Recipes

Basic Recipe I

1 Cup Epsom Salt

1/2 Cup Sea salt

1/4 Cup baking Soda

1/4 Borax

Basic Recipe II

1/2 cup Sea Salt

1/2 cup Magnesium flakes (these are easier to absorb)

1 Cup Epsom Salt

1/4 Cup Borax

Basic Recipe III (recommended for those with hypertension)

1 Cup Ground whole oats

1/2 Cup Magnesium Flakes

1/4 Cup Baking Soda

1/4 Cup Borax

Directions: Mix all the ingredients together before adding 1/4 cup into running Luke warm or slightly hot water.

You will need to mix these beforehand as they will need time to settle.

There are other ingredients you can add to the mixtures above to make the recipes therapeutic:

FROSTBITE/CHAPPED SKIN

I am talking about the early stages of frostbite. This is when your extremities are starting to lose feeling due to the cold. If you are outside too long and the symptoms worsen, you will need to see a doctor. Don't treat sever frostbite yourself.

1/4 ground Lavender Flowers

1/4 ground kelp

1/4 cup Spirulina

20 Drops Lavender Essential oil

20 Drops of Patchouli Essential oil (Excellent for chapped skin)

10 Drops of Geranuim Essential oil

1 Ounce of Sweet Almond or Apricot Seed oil

1 Ounce of Coconut oil

- Mix all the dry ingredients (including the recipe of your choice above) and set aside.

- Mix all of the liquid ingredients together.

  o You may need to melt the coconut oil, depending on how your thermostat is set in your home.

  o Most coconut oil stays solid at room temperature (75F)

- Slowly add the dry ingredients to the blend and place in an air-tight container overnight to allow all the ingredients to mix well.

MAINTENANCE BATH

2 ounces of Sweet Almond or Apricot Seed oil

20 Drops of Lavender essential oil

10 Drops of Roman Chamomile Essential oil

10 Drops of Geranium Essential oil

10 Drops of Peppermint Essential oil

- Mix all of these together

- Add the dry recipe of your choosing

Salt and Sugar scrubs

Finally, we get to the part of our skin we have tried everything we can think of to smooth out, our elbows and knees. Salt and sugar scrubs are excellent for exfoliation and helping to rid us of those unsightly patches of thick, tough skin. These will also work on the callouses of your feet.

The rule of thumb about how coarse the salt or sugar should be is determined by how rough and thick your patches are. If they are really rough, very coarse salt will do the trick. Do not apply these scrubs to broken skin. You will only make it worse.

BASIC SALT SCRUB RECIPE

1/2 Cup Sea Salt

1/2 Cup Epsom salt

1/4 Cup Borax

1/4 Cup and 3 tbsp Sweet Almond, Apricot seed, or Jojoba Oil

- Mix the dry ingredients before adding the oil.

- After mixing well, the salt should look wet and go on like a paste.

- Add just enough of the scrub to cover the area and allow to dry.

- Rewet it in the shower and scrub before removing.

- Follow-up by applying a plain carrier oil such as the ones listed above or Grapeseed oil

-

BASIC SUGAR SCRUB RECIPE

1/2 Cup Brown Sugar

3 tbsp Sweet Almond, Apricot Seed, or Jojoba Oil

- Mix all the ingredients together and use them as you would the salt scrub.

ALL-PURPOSE ESSENTIAL OIL BLEND FOR SCRUBS

For the salt scrub:

20 Drops Roman Chamomile Essential

10 Drops Lavender essential oil

5 Drops Geranium essential oil

For the sugar scrub, follow the ingredients in the order listed, but reduce it to the following:

10 Drops of the first one.

4 Drop each of the others.

General tips

Dress for the climate. In know this may seem elementary, but not dressing appropriately and staying covered in harsh winds and chilling weather can lead to your skin taking on a sick pallor and losing its elasticity. Frostbite can cause lost limbs and no one wants to lose a limb. Make sure what you are wearing protects your skin from the cold and the wind.

Moisturize your skin before leaving the house and again when you come after your shower or bath. This will help your skin retain moisture.

Drink plenty of fluids that hydrate you. Sodas and other carbonated beverages can dehydrate you and your skin due to the fact you're not getting enough liquid in your system.

For many of the recipes listed, you can just use the essential oil blends as body oil spot treatments to instantly soothe chapped and irritated skin.

If you have a favorite lotion, you can add an essential oil of your choice to boost its healing factor. The ratio for this is 6 drops per tablespoon of lotion.

You can also use that ration to add essential oils to existing shampoos and conditioners.

Conclusion

Winter is usually the harshest time of year. No one wants to go out, fearing freezing winds and temperatures that can freeze extremities, but it can't be avoided. Your home can be just as harsh because of your heating systems.

Using the tips and recipes in this book will help you control your dry skin and help prevent your hair from becoming brittle and having split ends. This book can also help you keep your skin looking moisturized and young.

Play around with the recipes and make some of your own. If you are not sure how, there are many reputable websites and forums on the internet that can help you with more recipes, advice, and encouragement.

Yes, winter can be harsh, but it doesn't have to be harsh on your skin.

FREE Bonus Reminder

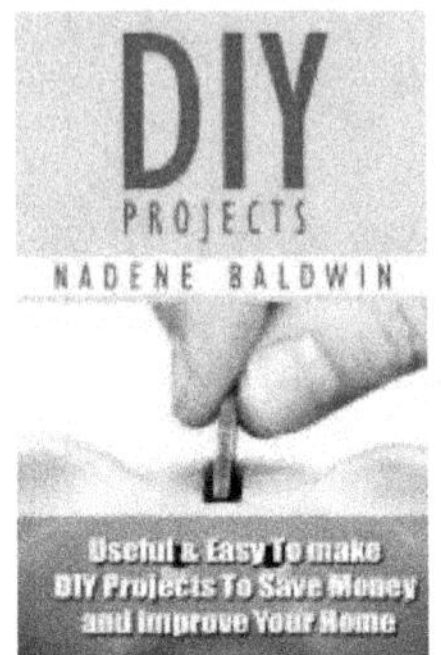

If you have not grabbed it yet, please go ahead and download your special bonus report *"DIY Projects. 13 Useful & Easy To Make DIY Projects To Save Money & Improve Your Home!"*

Simply Click the Button Below

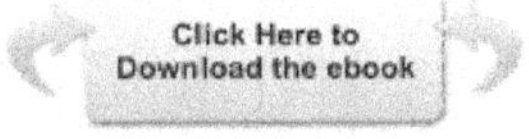

OR **Go to This Page**

http://diyhomecraft.com/free

BONUS #2: More Free & Discounted Books or Products

Do you want to receive more Free/Discounted Books or Products?

We have a mailing list where we send out our new Books or Products when they go free or with a discount on Amazon. Click on the link below to sign up for Free & Discount Book & Product Promotions.

=> Sign Up for Free & Discount Book & Product Promotions <=

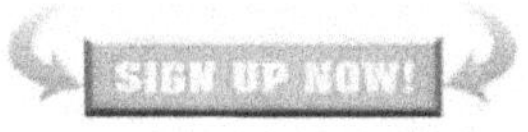

OR Go to this URL

http://zbit.ly/1WBb1Ek

www.ingramcontent.com/pod-product-compliance
Lightning Source LLC
Chambersburg PA
CBHW060823260726

48660CB00003B/1063